AF316784

THE

CHOCOLATE

DIET

HENRY H . PETERSOHN

ISBN : 979-8-3303-8044-2

Printed in United States Of America

Published by **Henry h . Petersohn**

Table of Contents

CHAPTER

01

01
WHY IS THE CHOCOLATE DIET SO SUCCESSFUL?

Chocolate is a favorite of many children and grownups. Sometimes we eat it in little bars or drops or pieces. Sometimes we have a drink of hot chocolate or coco or eat a piece of chocolate cake. Many times, chocolate is given to us on holidays like Christmas, Valentine's Day, Hannukah or our birthday. You can buy chocolates in a grocery store, a candy store and many other places. Unless your doctor has said NO, consider trying the

Chocolate Diet.

What should a chocolate diet involve? It needs to be a reasonably balanced diet so it should have lots of fresh fruit, vegetables, fish, chicken, eggs and some meat. This assortment of food is easily digested by the stomach and contains all the nourishment we need. A chocolate diet is much like a Mediterranean diet except for it's focus on eating small amounts of a dark chocolate bar as part of most desserts

CHAPTER

02

CHAPTER

03

02
WHY DOES THIS DIET WORK SO WELL?

Human beings eat a wide variety of foods in different quantities and at different times of the day. Fortunately, most of us have stomachs that are very adept in handling this situation. Actually, your stomach is a fantastic chemical processing operation that works 24 hours a day every day of your life and does this all in in a small space.

Regardless of the type of incoming food, the stomach produces a variety of enzymes and chemicals to dissolve that food and sends proteins, fat, vitamins, minerals and other food substances to the blood stream to nourish all the parts of the human body, and then sends left overs for disposal.

A baby starts with a tiny stomach that only has room for a few ounces of food. As a baby grows, it's stomach grows. An adult may easily be able to hold as much as a gallon or so in his stomach. Interestingly, when the stomach is not working, it squeezes itself down in size.

In contrast, food manufacturing plants in the world are generally much larger, fixed in size and typically focus on producing just a one or a few products. They also close down to allow frequent careful maintenance and are sometimes not working and need cleaning and repair.

03
WHAT CAN YOU EAT IF YOU ARE ON A CHOCOLATE DIET?

Most meals are almost the same as a typical Mediterranean style meal.

BREAKFAST.

There are several different breakfasts that work well for most people;

a) A bowl of oatmeal and some milk and a half a banana followed a chunk of several ounces of chocolate may work well for a real chocoholic.

b) A cup of hot chocolate made with milk along with two small handfuls of blackberries and two small handfuls of blueberries or blackberries and a half a banana works well for a small eater.

c) Some folks start with a minimum breakfast such as a bagel with cream cheese and a glass of orange juice. Make this breakfast healthier and tasty by also eating a fresh orange or a kiwi and adding a slice or two of smoked salmon (lox) to that bagel. That salmon tastes good and has both the good fish oil and the natural vitamin D your body needs. This is the same necessary

Vitamin D you could get from being in the sun but without the drying effects from the sun or sunburn. Add tea or coffee if you wish.

d) One popular breakfast is a few slices of crispy bacon over eggs with toast. Ouch! This tastes good but is not especially heathy. Make it better by adding a banana, a fresh orange, a kiwi or a handful or two of some fresh berries.

e) Many folks like stopping in a coffee shop and having a doughnut or pastry along with their drink. This can be an expensive habit that just stuffs you with fat calories that are not on any recommended diet. If you are watching your budget, be sure to add up the dollars. You may decide to spend your money on other things.

LUNCH

Lunch should be a lean Mediterranean style meal. If you like, add a bite of dark chocolate when you finish. Examples of lunch meals follow.

a) Try a large vegetable salad with an ounce or less of a dressing and some tuna fish or perhaps a hardboiled egg. Top It off with tea or coffee or just plain water.

b) Avocados - especially in the form of guacamole can be paired with some crackers or a slice of whole grain bread. Add a few small cherry tomatoes on the side to make a tasty lunch.

c) Chickpeas are a vegetable that many of us have seen in the form of humas. Chickpeas are high in protein and fiber plus Vitamin B6. Humus has a nice taste so it is often served as a dip for crackers or chips. For a nice quick and easy lunch, try it on a slice of whole grain bread and have a glass of low-fat milk. If you then want something sweet, take a few bites of dark chocolate.

d) For a different but easily made lunch, try sliced tomatoes on a slice of whole grain bread. Here is what you do. Take one or two slices of a crunchy bread such as a Harvest bread, lightly mayonnaise the bread, add a few grains of salt, and sprinkle it with black pepper. Now take a tasty small tomato. (I like Campari tomatoes because they are small, crunchy and keep well in a refrigerator). Slice a tomato and put the slices on the bread. This may be a little slippery to hold but just pop it into your mouth for a tasty treat.

e) Another good lunch at home is to open and eat a tin of sardines. Here we get the benefits of the natural oil in the fish. Whether packed in water, oil or mustard, sardines have lots of heart heathy fish oil, vitamins and minerals. Just open the tin and put the sardines on a piece of multigrain bread. Sardines are also a preferred seafood since their diet in the sea consists of very small creatures and natural items which means they have extremely low amounts of mercury. That's important since mercury, even in small amounts is a bad item for any human being. Pick up a few tins on your next shopping trip. These tins have a very long shelf life so it's easy to keep some on hand.

f) Freshly made pizza is always an easy appealing lunch, Try some with different toppings. i.e. sliced tomatoes, some pepperoni, perhaps some anchovies, mushrooms, etc. Wash the pizza down with a glass of water or iced tea.

g) Another good lunch is tuna salad or egg salad on a croissant, a kaiser roll or on some whole wheat toast. Skip having a coke or a pepsi and try ice tea instead.

h) Sometimes an omlet with a spoonful or two of cottage cheese is quite enough for a quick lunch.

DINNER

What about a Mediterranean style dinner? There are a number of excellent meals you can try. Many feature seafood. Some focus on pasta or eggs. Typical dinners would start with soup, then a salad - usually with one or another dressing, perhaps coleslaw, apple sauce, one or several common vegetables and a main course of fish, meat or possibly cheese plus a beverage.

Sometimes a precooked dinner will be brought in from a nearby restaurant, a grocery store or from a food takeout vendor. A favorite dinner is to bring in a whole roasted chicken. Often that take-out also includes some vegetables.

Many of the take-out vendors feature foods that are fried in oil – not in olive oil but generally in a not so good oil. French fries which so many of us like, are almost aways something to avoid. If you can't resist them, jut eat a few. Some examples of typically good dinner meals follow:

a) Fish. Try tilapia, salmon, trout or cod broiled with a drizzle of butter and served with a slice of lemon or a light sauce. Typical sides can include a salad such as lettuce, cucumbers, some pieces of mild onion rings, some sliced tomatoes and perhaps a little goat cheese.

b) Sometimes you would enjoy starting your dinner at home with a shrimp cocktail. Simply put 3-5 shrimp in a small dish and add some cocktail sauce.

c) Another way to start a tasty meal at a restaurant is to get a half dozen or more clams or oysters with the shells pried off and served to you on a bed of cracked ice. Eat the meat using some cocktail sauce and a few drops of lemon juice. That make them a real treat.

d) If you really enjoy fresh seafood, consider getting a pound or so of steamed mussels at a restaurant as your main course. Steaming them with garlic, lemon juice and wine opens their shells so you can pull the meat out.

e) Clams and oysters also make for a tasty clam chowder or a bisque.

f) Salmon is frequently the main course at dinner. When you think of salmon, the first thing to know is that it can be 'wild caught' in the sea or it could be grown in large closed ponds. In either case, it has a great deal of protein and some vitamins (Vitamin D) and other minerals that your body needs. It may be baked or broiled and often gets one of a half-dozen light sauces. The second interesting fact is that a great deal of salmon is smoked and is then known as lox. The bulk of this lox is then used with a smear of cream cheese to make a lox and bagel sandwich. This sandwich is often eaten at breakfast but tastes great at any time of the day.

g) A steak is often the major part of a dinner. Beef steaks are often fried. Since steaks are cut from different parts of a cow, they need to be cooked in slightly different ways to end up tasty and easy to chew. Common steaks are: strip steaks, skirt steaks, t-bone steaks, rib eye steaks and porterhouse steaks. In giving pieces of steak to small children, it is wise to keep them away from the very sharp steak knives and have an adult cut their steak into small pieces so they can easily chew the steak and not choke on a large chunk.

h) Lamb chops. This is a delightful meal for both adults and small children. It simply involves broiling some lamb chops. They are often served with some vegetables.

i) Another great beef dish is a pot-roast. This is a large piece of meat which has been roasted in an oven. This process tenderizes the meat and the potatoes, onions, carrots and the little bit of butter and flour you add creates a tasty gravy. Of course, one still need to cut up the serving you give to little children.

j) Ribs – Many people enjoy eating pork or beef ribs slathered with barbecue sauce. Pork ribs are generally smaller than beef ribs but both are popular at outdoor picknicks or at a fairground.

k) Kabobs – A kabob is a meal on a stick. It typically has chunks of chicken or beef with alternating chunks of tomatoes and green peppers all roasted on a stick. A kabob is easy for teenagers and adults to eat but one needs to take the food off the stick and cut it up for small children.

l) Chicken pot pie. This is a different type of hot meal where chicken, peas, carrots, onions and celery are cooked

together in a small serving cup and usually includes a
flaky crust.

m) A common favorite dinner meal is spaghetti and meat
balls in marinara sauce.Preparation is very similar both at
home and in a restaurant. Start by cooking dry spaghetti
for about 12 minutes in a microwave and then draining
it. Then open a quart jar of your favorite marinara sauce
(lots of choices on most grocery shelves). Heat the sauce
in a microwave-proof bowl - takes 3 to 4 minutes. Pour
the sauce on the spaghetti and add the cooked
meatballs. VOILA, If you have any left, it keeps well for a
few days in your refrigerator

DESSERTS

14

There are lots of desserts that people enjoy. On the top of the dessert list is chocolate in one form or another. There is often one or another type of chocolate cake, a brownie, chocolate cookies, a pudding cake or perhaps a Boston cream pie on that list. Two dessert lists follow. The first is a list of non-chocolate desserts. The second list is chocolate desserts.

NON-CHOCOLATE DESSERTS

Bread pudding

Cakes, Pies, Scones and Tarts made with all types of fillings and nuts

Apple, Cherry, Custard, Lemon Meringue, and Pecan pie are popular

Cheesecakes, often with different toppings, are a common favorite

Donuts are liked, but are more generally found as a breakfast or lunch treat

Fruits often appeaw as a dessert. Some common fruits include Apples, Bananas, Blackberries, Blue berries, Grapefruit, Grapes, Cantaloupes, Cherries, Oranges, KIWI, Peaches, Pears, Pineapples, Strawberries, Raspberries, Tangerines and Watermelon. In many instances, several kinds of fruit are mixed and served in a separate dish as a dessert

Nuts - Brazil Nuts, Cashews, Pecans, Pine Nuts, and Walnuts

Ice Cream is well liked and is often served with apple or cherry pie

Jello, Rice Pudding

CHOCOLATE DESSERTS

You need a chocolate diet that revolves around dark chocolate bars. They not only taste very good but have a number of very important health benefits for you. Some dieticians claim that an 85% cacao content dark chocolate bar is especially tasty and also has less sugar than regular milk chocolate.

People like the taste of dark chocolate bars and enjoy eating them which immediately reduces stress and feelings of anxiety.

Dark chocolate bars are rich in powerful antioxidants and healthy fats that combat damage caused by free radicals that contributes to aging, heart disease, cancer, Alzheimer's and other diseases. At the same time, they can reduce a person's normal level of insulin resistance, and slow down the absorption of sugar into the bloodstream thus lowering blood pressure and reducing the risk of stroke and heart disease.

Components of the cocoa bean and it's fatty acids in dark chocolate bars also help protect the skin against the harmful effects of UV light by increasing boost blood flow, helping your skin look better and also helping your skin stay hydrated.

Dark chocolate contains magnesium, manganese, copper, zinc and phosphorus, all of which build bones. It boosts blood flow in the brain which also helps minimizes dementia and strokes.

CHAPTER

04

04
HURRAH FOR DARK CHOCOLATE

Do you know how we found out about chocolate and started using it? It actually started in Mexico where the seeds grow on small coco trees. These seeds were dried and turned into beans. The first people to pick these coco beans were an ancient Indian group known as Aztecs. They roasted the beans, then ground and squeezed them into coco butter and drank the bitter stuff since hey believed that chocolate made them better warriors and more manly. Explorers in Mexico brought the beans back to Europe. Then a Dutch chemist found a way to make the beans into a coco powder and then extracted the coco butter. That butter could then be mixed with sugar and milk to make a cup of sweet, tasty hot chocolate. Wealthy people in Europe tried this hot chocolate it and liked it very much. Soon, many shops in Europe started making chocolate bars and chocolate candies. Even today, much very good chocolate is made in Europe. The United States, England, Germany and Switzerland also make very good chocolate.

It is estimated that 1 <u>billion</u> people eat chocolate every day so it's no surprise to discover there are at least 20 - 40 brands - many marketed in across the world - each with claims of being the greatest. Often well-known brands are marketed as premium priced items – although less expensive brands may taste just as well – or better for you. Some of the better-known brands include: Cadbury. Hotel Chocolate, House of Dorchester, Galaxy (England), Nestle, Toblerone, Lindt (Switzerland), Hershey, Ghirardelli (United States), Moser Roth, Choceur (German), and Godiva (Belgian). Several brands including Hershey, Moser Roth, and Choceur are carried at heavy price discounts by the well-known ALDI grocery chain.

A recent study from Consumer Reports was printed by the New York Post The study specifically identified well known brands which had dangerous amount of cadmium, lead or both as well as chocolate that had very low levels of these chemicals. Godiva Signature Dark, Hershey Special Dark Mild, Lindt Excellent Dark, Dove Premium Deep Chocolate and Trader Joe's Dark chocolates were found to have dangerous levels of cadmium and lead. Brands that had low levels included Ghiradelli Intense Dark Chocolate and less popular brands.

THANK YOU